Homo Invitus

Homo Invitus

MEMOIRS OF A GENIE

Ngong Margretson

To order additional copies of this book, contact:
Xlibris Corporation
0-800-644-6988
www.Xlibrispublishing.co.uk
Orders@Xlibrispublishing.co.uk
301930

For positives and negatives, they are no longer seating on the fence.

Memoirs are penned at the twilight of supposedly Jekyll careers. Mine paints Mr. Hyde, a dawning in a dusk quest. You will read it because it marks your house for my Passover . . . that is if you heed. Many will not admit to the existence of a devil unless they get a direct confession. Here is a dare devil's confession and absolution.

Chapter One

THE FAST LANE

I am listening to the steady beep-beep coming from the sophisticated machine at the Medical Emergency Unit (MEU) of the National Hospital, Abuja. At the back of my absent mind I know it would sooner than later transform into a "dirge" continues tune. That is because I've been doing more than passive listening. The case fatality of life is one hundred percent. Everybody surely dies, I know. But I decimate the life expectancy of those I assail. I execute the family business with unparalleled diligence; I follow up each task to an illogical conclusion.

I was here to facilitate a couple's demise years ago when these machines came in. I'd overheard Dr. Whaler, the consultant physician, boasting how they were state of the art, imported from Germany. All his resident doctors were to be acquainted with them. Residents and patients listen to him. He was good . . . still good, but not good enough for me. You see he is medical, I am methodical. My strike is critical, his is clinical. He extorts and inhibits my virulence while I extol and exhibit my violence. The couple went to the great beyond, the machines stayed for the next patient.

A battle won and lost, a debacle still raging hot.

I strayed invincibly to prey on my next victim.

The Hospital is an ultra modern edifice built initially as the National Hospital for Women and Children by the Abacha junta. It has grown to represent the benchmark for medical practice in the nation. However, other peripheral clinics are on the verge of converting it into a mega-death row. They keep my victims, suck up their remaining monies while I suck the life out of them, and then refer them in, knowing I am hot on their trail to finish the job. Most patients are therefore triaged death—my illogical conclusion.

The MEU suite 1 is six bedded, each usually with a patient and a story that has been well researched and catalogued in the light brown folders on the desk. About four reviews are entered per patient, each continually refined to precision by the next tier in the medical hierarchy, from the rookie through the Residents to the Consultants and professors. Today my jurisdiction is limited to Moses here—it's all there in the folder labelled Moses Ali. They are days I have all six beds to myself with some spill over to the next suite.

I am here to feel him breathe his last. He only needs a nudge now. I mustn't be the one prodding but I am here anyway; the arch-wrath master acting his wretch art with no spare wreath arc. He knows I am waiting and he too can't wait for the death knell beep that he would barely hear. Killing is now a healing euthanasia. He waits to exhale into oblivion as I excel. I can see he is gone past caring, he is caving in. I know I am gone past cheering, I am sneering out.

My guillotine bids hither.

He is a mesh of wires, tubes and limbs that look like bigger tubes abutting the drained tank of a torso. They is a pipe up his left nostril, two in the mouth, one emanating from his now baggy trouser and one from the back of each frail hand. I understand some brought food, air and other, fluids.

None is taking me or my effect away. I am the super. I am in control.

He has six wire contacts on his chest wall, has every limb clasped by a bright colour coded plastic tong—red, yellow, green and black. A cuff is wrapped round his left arm and another devise stuck to his thumb. These feed Whaler's machines and monitors above. The "toys" keep an eye on my progress as he regresses. So far, none of them is making me less comfortable. These and the white sheet are the only normal entities around this man who has degenerated into less than an object of ridicule. The nurse's excellent job of cleaning him unveiled a dramatic arithmetic expression of bossing` bones, parched shrunken semitransparent skin and sunken eyeballs that fall short of transmitting to a whole being.

To the medical community and its luminaries, I blatantly ask. "Is that the best that you could come with?"

You can see something is grossly wrong but you don't see any hideous gunshot wounds or haemorrhaging gash typical of other assassin's work. The surgeons have no bleeders to catch and fix; the physicians have no sure bet aliquots to dole. Any hope of recovery is farfetched and if attainable can be a slow process reminiscent of the long time I took to goad him to this precipice. Whaler can showcase his clinical acumen and sophistication, the patient can have some dignity, your so called advanced life support and combined anti retroviral therapy, but too late, he will still wind down dead to my marksmanship. That's me at my hype. It is a trademark I am proud of.

The night duty nurse hovers around, peering through thick lens to the monitor above. She looks down at the emaciated gasping wired figure and shakes her head disparagingly. The strung out figure reminds her of a spider, ironically stuck on its web, sucked and grilled by the silky self-made grid.

I brace myself. Orgasm is almost here, the funk fun almost over.

"Pulse oximeter reading 61% on 13 litre oxygen?" She declares solemnly. "Agonal rhythm on electrocardiogram." This deterioration did not surprise her as the good doctor had listed him in "critical condition" this afternoon. To those who knew Dr. Whaler, that statement was a death sentence. The poor guy was a goner. The doctor knew I was done with the man and he was done for.

A House Officer clad in saintly white ward suit loiters around; the last line of defence left behind to fight and eventually surrender the patient to me. He would be needed to certify my success. He wills the machine to give the last shrill beep, the so called whistle of death, so he too can proceed to those without his boss's "death sentence". He has his dead certification lines memorized. He had done it so many times it had become a ritual. That wasn't surprising; he was on my epicentre, which meant he would still write out those medical farewell lines severally:

"Called to review patient whose respiratory efforts had ceased.
Two wide bore lines in place dispensing *normal saline.*
Oro-tracheal tube and a *pharyngeal airway* in place.
ECG showing an iso-electric line.
Cold clammy extremities noted.
No spontaneous respiratory effort observed.
No cardiac activity detectible.
Pupils are dilated, fixed and non reactive to light.
Assessment: Clinically death."

Then the time of demise will be inserted with an addendum informing the relatives and the morgue. That was the easy part. The waiting was the hard part. But it would surely happen this night . . . it happened. In my domicile—his bloodstream, I could feel the gradual sludge to a halt. I could hear the long beep. I could feel the hideous cold engulf me.

The doctor didn't have to wait any longer. The nurse waves frantically and he dutifully walks over almost thankfully.

No resuscitation was in the offing. For my moribund victims, resuscitation is almost unmerciful. I have slowly slipped a *Do Not Resuscitate* order into most clinician's psych. That leaves only palliation on the table. Nurse Theresa is already shutting down the hopeless Omron monitor and with it the petulant beep. The time is 20:42. That's how far Moses made it, the rookie notes.

Nurse Theresa mumbles a prayer committing the soul of the faithfully departed to her God. I wondered whether Moses Ali had been a faithful. It is unnecessarily assumed that my victims are not.

The rookie takes the case notes to document my pyrrhic victory. All is silent. Death silences even me, but unlike my victims, in this silence, I do have other salient advantages of proliferation.

I do not know if or when I was born. But I have long figured out why. If I were to have a résumé, my occupation and hobby would read "killing." I would give a unisex name. Not because I loathe sex—I thrive on it. I would be ageless with an infinite life expectancy.

Millions of people have been trying to pick my brain but have failed woefully because I don't seem to have one. And yet somehow I am no dimwit. I say this confidently because given my conquest to size ratio, I can arrogantly add the prefix genius to my feared genie name.

I have killed innumerably. Men, women, children, young, old, rich, poor, I do them all. I have wiped out families and clans. The good, the bad, the ugly, I don't discriminate. It's horrendous justice at a tremendous pace.

People are more afraid of me than the death I transpose. I have featured in a couple of suicide notes. Funny, I am on my way to the kill and my victim decides and helps me out. Some will rather die in silence than raise an alarm that could salvage them. They procrastinate until I become a red herring that can't be undone. Eventually they end up with cold clammy extremities, stoppage of heart activity and breathing, dilated fixed pupils—like poor Moses here, they expire.

I don't have a count. The world has lost its count. Last time they checked, they claimed I had killed twenty five million and counting. I agreed with the counting part. I argued the quoted meagre number. They also estimate I am on to at least forty million and recruiting an alarming five thousand daily. Yes, I am cramming my boundless arena with gladiators and you can already hear them hail, "We who are about to die, salute you!"

I have infected plenty and affected all. I affect you as you read my gory tale. I lurk around knocking for you to open a door or a window. When I get one, I come in almost peacefully to orchestrate your demise. Then I idly watch you deteriorate. Leer as people try this and that, blaming black and white powers. At this juncture, I lose interest in you and focus on those others, hoping they will make a mistake I can capitalise on.

I am pissed at this hospital and mundane Abuja. Sometimes their meticulousness shuts me out. Not even a crack for me. Bad manners, no one asks me in these days. Some even try asking me out. Some eat their cake and have it because Dr. Whaler has given them some of my secrets. He doesn't know them all. Nobody knows all about me. Not even my conceited self. The more rural knows less and I capitalize on lack of knowledge. To me, there is no excuse for the absence of knowledge. In such scenario, I usurp so much power. What's more, I can be in so many places at the same time. It's not like I am beating my own drum, but what assassin snipes multiple targets at the same instance, killing multiply at the same time? The worst of murderers think of serial killing, but I introduced parallel killing on a wide scale—a feat more than a shade away from the imaginations of *Holly*—and *Nollywood*. But that's my trait. The careless ones are my treat and I am a threat to the family, national and international security. That is understating it. I am the enemy within.

I wasn't always this strong and popular but every dog's got its day. These are my days, my decades and I am making the most of it. Believe me I am on a global spree. Because they can't kill me they have resorted to looking for my roots . . . taproots is the right word. They figure this could bring them closer to knowing me better and someday go for the kill. It's a long shot that seems to be working for me instead. The languages are now plenty. Theories, hypothesis, fables . . . you name them. I am the hub of so many conspiracies and controversies. What happened when mankind tried to build the tower of Babel is happening all over again. Only now I am the god that has cast the disuniting spell. Mr. A says I have a dark demeanour, supported by his computers and history he declares me indigenous to Africa. No, Mr. B thinks my lethality points to a Western creation. The finger pointing continues as Mr. C disagrees with other folks. He is religious and asserts I was created, like every other thing by his God.

I laugh and then I gloat. I don't believe in that kind of god. I can't. You shouldn't if you believe he created me to do what I do.

In a way, they are all correct as I will soon explain. I have patches of my story. Not all. I can't say for sure when I became a being but I do know when I started killing. I also know I had a peaceful coexistence in dense vegetations with animals. Monkeys, gorillas, cats, cows, I lived commensally with. I did not have the blueprint for the big killing league. I was with lower Primates, while you pre-empted me to pyramid to the real primate. My promotion was hatching. I was primed.

The CIA, FBI, MOSSAD, M-I5, CDC, UNICEF, FSB, UN, NSA, OAU and WHO were blind to my ingenious threat (in espionage, I hear talks of double agents; me, I have infiltrated all these agencies).

Why will I now declare an all and out war on people? What did they ever do to me? I know I don't sound like your average killer with no conscience. I am not your average killer. Sometimes I wish I was. My reputation precedes me and it shouldn't.

I lost it. I recall being swept off in an avalanche of "come and kill me" chorus from a choir that was the world. My invitation to the kill had arrived. From then it was easy. My effects were famous even when I was not known. The patient dog had earned the farthest fattest bone. It was time for the fastest chew—an ambitious churning chew of humanity.

*   *   *

Now let me pause to blab again. I probably have been to every country on planet earth. I have registered my presence in all your adorned cardinal points. It's been pressured business during my client's pleasure rendezvous. I have preyed on Muslims as they prayed and thronged around their Holy Kabba, I have been doused with Holy water at St. Peter's Basilica by none other than his Holiness, Pope John Paul the second of blessed memories. I have also had holy showers from his successor, all with no attendant miracles. I have dined on the Archbishop of Canterbury's table and I'm still hungry. I have been to Aso Rock under the military junta to the lucky guy's democratic government; to the White House when it was white and when it tanned, to 10 Downing Street long before Brown put in his resignation letter for Cameron to form a new government. Seen so many changes around and still stuck around without changing. Respect me and give me a personality befitting my status. I am the big boss and can be real bossy if you allow me.

I have been within target distance of all the big dudes you can think of, fair enough the small dudes too. But I am a special one. I need more than your usual target distance. You will think this reduces my prowess. Think again. I have access to the most wanted men on earth. Again, you will think the US will have me whack people like Osama. Again think again. I don't work for the US. I am my own man. I am even more wanted than that laden bin of terrorism, which means if you had one sure slug that could do away with one of us, even the US will gun for me in lieu of Osama. They are spending millions of Dollars to find him and now he can barely move, whereas they know where I reside and have dedicated billions to curb me and it doesn't even scare me. I am not just Houdini; I am in a class of my own. I am a titan. I am small and ubiquitous, yet my spread and stealth astounds. Did you know I was on both planes that named and maimed 9/11. And I am here to tell the story. Who else is? I am that good. I was the one that killed . . . No! I shouldn't be calling names. It's classified. Even the family doesn't want the grim details. The case stays hush—unsolved. The preferable phrase "brief illness" takes my exalted place.

I think big things even while doing some small ones. For instance I wish I could infiltrate and kill people like Mandela. I wish I killed Magic Johnson decades ago. That would have removed the Magic from his name. I wish I beat Parkinson and old age to the late Pope and mother Theresa respectively . . . Now that will be some news, wouldn't it? Shush, my big mouth, my big travels and my big skilled kills. It seems Mandela knows that only Mandela can allow me to kill Mandela. I admit it makes me powerless. But not everyone is Mandela and perhaps everyone can be *a* Mandela. Magic Johnson kept his magic by not hiding me; people can keep their karma by emulating him. The Pope and mother Theresa kept their distance respectably and earned my respect and respite. People should learn from them.

The Sherlock that fetched me out was this intelligent and dedicated dude. It was a cold day in May 1983 in the United States of America. I was doing several jobs in parallel and series. This whiz kid sniffed me out after a lengthy stake out. I'd been callous and careless since the summer of 1981. Many people had seen my work and he knew where and how to look. I had it coming while I had it going. He blew my cover.

In a historic press conference, he gave the startling decelerating declaration naming me the perpetrator behind the mass parallel and serial murders. It wasn't just a news flash. It generated a reverberating buzz in the media. The world stood at its feet. Every one raised a hand for a throat squeeze. Everyone screamed the death sentence. He was the hero, I was the villain. His forensic lab had dug hard enough to be infallible. He had just the evidence to nail me and I lacked an exonerating alibi.

Apparently, he'd opened Pandora's Box. Suddenly, I was being linked to jobs I'd forgotten. Asia and my renowned epicentre, Sub Saharan Africa, rang as often as jingle bells in the yuletide. My sins were glaring. I had to fry. A pound of my flesh was in high demand.

Then there was the brawl between the bounty hunters on who gets the accolades for the grab. Apparently, some Holmes French kid had pointed me out months earlier. This pitched the French against the American camp in a war of rhetoric that irked even their English/French translators. Finally, a truce that gave credit to both Mr. Sherlock and Monsieur Holmes was called.

They were still reeling in the shock discovery of the nonentity whodunit, when I pled guilty and sent the next shockwaves. The plea was with a brazen message that I was impenitent and will go scot-free to kill again and again (if my editor had allowed me "and again" would have reverberated for pages), same trademark pattern—multiple, slow, painful, parallel and serial. With six billion vulnerable people out there, I had a long list to prey on. My signature would be indelible. It already was. Even world wars gaped in awe.

And so the world stood still as the glare of an unrepentant unstoppable manslayer hit every blind spot. What was more? They had asked for a pound of flesh and they were damn well going to take it, exactly a pound, no more, no less. No blood spilled. Smart merchant of the universe, I hear you muse.

Now, isn't that daring? How can I be this defiant? How can I show no remorse? Wasn't I forcing the judge to send me to death row? I can afford to be defiant. You can't. Remorsefulness is not in my dictionary. 1983 is like three decades away, and I am still here. It's been a long time in my death row but you are the ones suffering, dying and weeping. I still supervised this last guy go. My penchant for the kill game hasn't ebbed one bit, if anything it has stepped up some notches.

People make me kill them. People sign the contract for me to whack them. I am at your beck and call to whack you. I rarely accept proxy contracts or contacts. If it is any consolation or consolation, the good old days of clandestine killings are gone. I am no longer invisible, but the good old killing is still on. I am still invincible. Sadly for me, people have more ways of keeping me at bay now. The likes of Dr. Whaler are putting up a good fight. I guess that drew the thin line between kill or be killed.

A pity, the quake I wrought is so heart quirking it can't be measured by your Richter scale and since I can't move the epicentre, I plan to implode. Here now, is how you get a safe haven. The world's most prolific killer is letting you in on modus operandi secrets that guarantee permanent restraining orders. The incredible accounts of a small time criminal mind with mammoth ambitions, a supporting system to piggyback on, rear a mere iceberg tenth of the effect, with the damaging chunk hidden beneath the cold murky waters.

It has been obituaries, mortuaries and no sanctuaries for Africa warranting this mayday call from mayhem to Mayfair. I hope it removes Africa's future from my blood thirsty clutch.

Chapter Two

THE ORIGIN

Time stood still for her at six a.m. Miss Cyan was not just waking up. She had not slept one bit. She yawned and stretched tiredly on the stale linen clad divan. She was tired from a night of harder work. I knew because I was in her shabby little den from dusk to dawn. I don't think the man who brought me knew he had just served as my courier. He didn't act suspicious as he delivered the package in style saving his fair share. For the barely twenty three year old prostituting destitute, it had been all work and no play but it was worth it. She was twenty thousand naira richer and an OTC analgesic would put her in the clear—or so she thought. In Nigeria twenty thousand could buy you a slave for a month. She had been more than just a slave for a month contracted into one gross Saturday night. It was a fast buck at stake. Despite the sores on various orifices, I saw the gleam as she stretched her mouth to sketch a smile on her face when the money changed hands.

It was a quality—quantity tussle. What you guys will call "off the hook" and be happy about. That man had a banality of carnal, oral and anal knowledge of this woman—a lot of leeway for me if you ask. She had endured most part of, and survived to enjoy briefly, the twenty thousand naira stipend.

I heard her feigned pleasure that was actually pressure all night. I heard his groans as he ejaculated again and again and all I had to do was to get a good grip for the attaching attack.

Now I am here. My vigil has started for both of them. Technically speaking, for him it started two years ago.

With my modus operandi, arithmetic progression of victims is the past and geometric progression is an enviable future. Every index job has at least, another one on standby. By the time I am done with Cyan, she would have conscripted even more to my cause. That is why I allow a long dutiful vigil. And that is why I do not agree with your much publicized phrase; "brief illness."

Cyan was beautifully built but her self-afflicted finishing was furnished off beam. The hair was clearly not legit. The off coloured tresses trickled down a face almost disguised with makeup that didn't make up. However, once the lights were dimmed—as they had been throughout the night, the silhouette was superb. Chubby round moaning face, chubby round succulent breast, chubby round cushioning buttocks, chubby round clasping labia and the chubby round song could go on and on in any masculine philharmonic. These did not appeal to me but I'm sure all this went through the man's mind and kept reinvigorating him all night or he had probably taken a couple of those blue pills. Good thing for me, his libido was this good and she wasn't about to lose her bait features just yet. She is my newest Petri dish, one of the formidable weapons at my disposal waiting invitingly for my covert proliferation bids. It will take months to years for the world to know I have marked her for death and its appendages. The real damage would have been done.

The man was well built and insisted on "skin to skin". No condoms . . . sucking a candy with a gloved tongue wasn't that appealing, he mumbled. This raised her bargaining power.

I licked my lips. If only she knew.

When he left, I lapsed into one of my reprisal vigil. Were they ever going to curb me? When I was discovered, I thought that was about the moribund of my loathed career. How wrong I was. Yes, they have been some deceleration in my kill rate. Some became wiser as I was further elucidated. But it appears the jury wasn't that unanimous. Some other faction suddenly claimed that I was a figment of Western imagination. They argued that I did not exist and wasn't responsible for the perpetuating holocaust. To think after my feat, they could still be a sane soul that did not acknowledge me. I felt insulted but the news was good for business. My gravy train sped on.

I am notorious for getting and never forgetting sexual tourists, customers that drink too much alcohol, smoke too much hash, listen to loud music, hyper socializes, and do drugs especially intravenously. These are the folks that keep the vogue that keeps me in vogue. They furnish the appropriate "fun" for me to patch on an "eral" suffix. I am allured by their invitation. With a fatal handshake, I come in and put them into more misery before helping them out of it for good. Everyone is a potential client, straights and gays alike. From the spoils of the pools and pits to the finesse of pulpits and the drabness of culprits, the caves, the mansions, Guantanamo bay, you name them, not even a mother's womb is a safe haven. I laud polygamous settings, because it makes it easier for me to move freely with so many targets in my line of fire.

People, as you may well know, have continued the heated debate as to my origin and emergence as a global economic force to reckon with. I am sure you have one version you agree with. I have mine too. While some religious proponents ascribe me to a divine punishment on the race for its waywardness, the West is of the opinion that I came from Central Africa. Others remain adamant that I am a biologic warfare agent created by the West to stem a teeming third world populace. Some even claim the killings are just not connected. They say they are multi-factorial and I am just a political gimmick created in peoples mind to take the fall. And in the grassroots of Africa, some people are still oblivious of my existence even as I move within in carnage! I wince when I hear a new theory and I sum up your speculations to get mine. You guys are smart. But I am smarter.

Patches of logical evidence elevate these hypotheses from mere conjectures in the eyes of their faithful followers. I pause to listen as these intelligent beings bicker. For example, religious proponents are of the opinion that man has strayed far away from his creator with more sins, yet unheard of being committed. They cite the legalization of abortion in some countries, euthanasia, gay marriages, gay priest and man on the verge of making man in the art of cloning as enough reason for God to hit back in time to stem man's attempt to build another tower of Babel. The conspiracy theorist maintains that the United States, in a mad drive for alternative warfare supremacy after failing to curtail nuclear proliferation, inadvertently created and unleashed a new lethal force—me. The Afro-origin proponents, presently the most accepted, base its claim on computer studies, my existence around some African primates and the fact that some of my hits were traced back to Africa. Ever heard of slims disease? My own theory: they are all correct.

Not so fast. They are loopholes blighting these theories. For instance, a creator as divine as the one they call God would not hurl such a killer on his creation. Especially not one so illogical that it could strike sinner and saint alike, thereby punishing the innocent and allowing some guilty ones to escape by using some candour umbrella, pompously and purposefully given out by people like Dr. Whaler and blasphemously elevating the condom's status to an innovative modern day Noah's ark. On the other hand, the United States would not author and disseminate a killing machine that will place such a meteoric burden on itself—the fight against me even in sub Saharan Africa is substantially funded by the United States. Again, if as the West opine, I had a humble origin from apes, why did the apes seem to play the host more comfortably whereas I deal mercilessly with man? It seems all these theories have only spawned a sense of limbo, generated and fuelled more misconceptions about my humble self. It's time I quelled the glowing controversies from growing. Buckle up scholar, I am about to get scientific and cerebral on you. Follow my lead.

*   *   *

I envisaged a unifying theory that incorporates all the others and allows you to concentrate on the future and consecrate the past. I dubbed it *Man's Irrational Selection Tsunami* theory or simply, the *MIST* theory. It's just a thin film off the fog created by the gamut of rioting theories that makes up this mystifying "mist" of mine.

I will spool back to a hundred and fifty years, when I was still in the wilds. Charles Darwin propounded the most acceptable theory of evolution. Natural selection and the survival of the fittest summed it up. My MIST theory views my humble self as an unleashing of Darwin's anger on your race for its gross disregard for his survival of the fittest principle. Every living thing has obeyed this principle except of course, man. While plants and animals struggled to survive at the mercy of Darwinism, you annihilated natural selection and indulged on a spree of irrational selection creating an unhealthy scenario of a survival of both the fittest and the un-fittest and consequently filled the earth with both cabbage and garbage.

I envied you as you swaggered from caves to mansions, invaded space and gallivanted on the moon, scaled Everest, dived and dined under the sea. You had sex with man and probably animal. With hi-tech installations like laminar flow theatres coupled with heroic surgeries, cardiac pacemakers, renal and cardiac transplantation, respirators, fourth and fifth generation antibiotics, vaccines, in-utero fertilization and in-utero surgeries, you sidelined natural selection allowing naturally selected to die "unfit" and "un-fittest" to survive and propagate. You also created feasible platforms for even the "fittest" to be exterminated. This did not probably go down well with the bearded theorist's ghost as it allowed such "misfits" to perpetuate the reason for their negative natural selection and gave room for some fitting lineages to be forever lost. I moved from the wild cabbage to the deadly domestic garbage by the same mechanism. I became, in effect, a knuckle of Darwin's fist of fury.

I am a by-product of an evolutionary trend truncated by an otherwise well meaning human endeavour, an untoward effect of your civilization. I have my roots in your modification of the natural selection process by unnatural means thereby creating a system fraught with mismatched pairs. Natural selection would have as it has in some lower animals, evolved Homo sapiens that would have hosted me at less peril than the conundrum you now have in my killing expedition. Having been able to influence your evolutionary spectrum, you eliminated the innate temporal evolution of your being and allowed "misfits" to thrive and provide a fertile milieu for the evolution of newer threatening entities. These "unfits" served over time as Petri dishes for newer scenarios to which even your "fittest" were naïve.

My theory laments that the field of human endeavour, backed (or hacked) by modern civilization has achieved a rather pyrrhic and untenable victory over Darwinism and sort of instituted a social Darwinism. Therefore, those who are not privileged these unnatural selection etiquettes are slowly phased out while those that can afford it are aided and abated despite inherent flaws. It means that we may well be slowly losing the "fittest" while the "unfit" are increasing with dire cumulative consequences of which I may just be the tip of the iceberg. Hence, in the long run what would have been a contained endemic in a population of more "fits" than "unfits" would rapidly degenerate into a pandemic in a reverse cohort.

Here is what obtains with your irrational selection. Those who can't afford properly screened blood for transfusion, funds or insurance coverage for drugs or say a kidney transplant, education on conduct or even a condom for that matter, are subconsciously socially selected as "unfit" and hence candidates for annihilation. On the contrary, for those who can afford these, you have pitched your technological might against natural selection. When an entity like me goes haywire, a massacre is the outcome because the ratio of the "fit" to the "unfit" has been reduced by the industrialized nation's multitude of medically sustained individuals and the increased mortality of even the "fit" through wars, poverty, natural disasters and other inventions of man. Imagine, for instance, how many "fit" or "fittest" died in 9/11 or in the Rwandan genocide.

Haven't you noticed that all things being equal, I tend to proffer a better prognosis when I work where natural selection abounds than where irrational selection flourishes? Read up HIV-1 and 2. Then what will you say if I told you of the phenomenon noticed in Kenya and The Gambia. They are a select group of people I have actually had in direct line of fire who seem to be immune to me. I have actually gotten into some people and found it hard or taken much longer to enact my act. Would these represent the descendants of those that toed the line of Darwinism? Would everyone have been like them had Darwinism prevailed? Would I have remained cabbage?

I am no doubt unique. No one could have created me in a lab—not even the great United States. As a matter of fact, I am mad at them. They represent the focal custodians of this irate selection I just described and decried. I actually set out on a mission to lay the west to rest in the waste of my wake. But unlike the typical African who can be many things from homosexual to HIV positive and hoard/hide it, these people are open about me; they made and took drugs thereby shifting my sting. They evaded me by eliminating to the barest minimum, poverty and ignorance. Lastly, only a god would plague me on his creation and Apes could only have bequeathed me to humanity through the evolutionary process. I have always been around. Man rather precipitated my actions by presenting a weaker race through his irrational selection of the "unfit" and occasional de-selection of the "fittest".

Conclusively, I know the West is only at fault for unleashing me because it undermined natural selection with its "tsunami" of medical and technological knowhow, nurturing the "unfit" to survive the perceived Darwinian onslaught as well as creating a world that could waste even the healthiest and relatively spare the wealthiest. Religion is at fault for limiting the use of proven methods to keep me at bay and allowing polygamous marriages in which a single target has potentially far reaching consequences. You are at fault if you have not checked for my presence or if you discriminate when I am found. My dissidents could just be a shade away from being correct; I would not necessarily have killed had natural selection prevailed! The finger pointing and disinformation surrounding my origin must henceforth be laid to rest in the *MIST* theory lest your pain remain my champagne.

It is however pertinent to stress that unlike the universe, I had no singular "Big Bang" but rather an evolutionary conditional progression from subtypes, which therefore precludes a straightforward lone "Big Crunch". It means that even more technological advancement and breakthrough (unfortunately more unnatural selection) is warranted to contain me. Humanity must also seek to curb wars, plane, train and industrial accidents and other arenas through which the world is being depleted of its "fittest".

I occasionally wonder if man can outwit Darwinism by modifications cautioned with mortification. I am that covert bullet ricocheting around your globe, splashing death throes and making homes death rows. You can drop the speculations, look the facts over and make informed decisions. Fair enough, that is your chance to get far away from the bloodbath.

Chapter Three

THE SELLOUT

1.   Write a HIV-AIDS article for my desk cleaner's consumption.

I ran tumultuous eddies in his bloodstream and so could read his mind. It was a trick question, he deciphered. On one hand, it was compulsory and carried a higher score; on the other hand they were still four more essay type questions to be answered from five—all in two hours. He looked at his wristwatch and mentally allocated a time frame for each question. "Thirty minutes tops, twenty each for the remaining four and ten minutes for review." He muttered. He had to be precise and straight to the point using very little medical mumbo-jumbo since it was intended for a semi-literate. The temptation was great to go writing down everything he had learned about this virus he had fallen prey to at a tender age of twenty six and thereby risk faring badly in other questions.

He was a final year medical student at the renowned University of Maiduguri Teaching Hospital. He had amassed a great deal of knowledge about the disease. The ink flowed freely as he told his Professor's desk cleaner about me. That I, a member of the *Lentivirus* (characterized by a long latent phase) family, was discovered in 1983 and established a year later as the agent behind the popular ailment called Acquired

Immune Deficiency Syndrome. He did not delve much on how I came to be. He didn't believe in the accepted theory of his native Africa being the source. He would however note the epidemiological data of my brunt describing it as being felt more in sub-Saharan Africa and Asia by writing out the estimated statistics with regards deaths, incidence and prevalence, expatiating that this was only a tip of the iceberg. Data collection was not good around here and they was a lot of bias in the reporting.

He wrote that I was transmitted mainly through sexual routes emphasizing heterosexual transmission in his locality. He'd know . . . that was how I got to him in the first place. He then went on to delve on homosexual, blood transfusion, vertical transmission (mother to child), needle stick injury and IV needle sharing. He added a note about holding hands, eating together, hugging, cough and mosquito bites not constituting a transmission risk.

He told the hypothetical medically layman that once I got into the system, I mainly attacked the immune system depleting special cells called Clusters of Differentiation 4(CD4) cells thereby rendering the body systems defenceless. He didn't irk them with the various stages of viral replication but explained that I hijacked the cellular processes for my purported evil purposes.

He described the new HIV positive patient the way he would describe himself: usually asymptomatic. Some presented with enlarged lymph nodes before going into the latent stage he presently was in. At the other extreme, he described various disease conditions that late comers usually presented with. I am sure he meant the likes of Moses Ali.

He delved on the all important concept of opportunistic infections in which disease conditions that a good immune system would have sorted become rife and life threatening because of my overwhelming presence. At the end of the gory spectrum he defined some AIDS defining conditions stating that it wasn't the lot for those diagnosed earlier. He added a note on AIDS related malignancies. He also said this clinical spectrum correlated with the CD4 count and went on to classify clients into A, B and C depending on the count.

For diagnosis, he stressed that earlier was better, he didn't add that he was a living testimony to this. He advocated for a yearly voluntary counselling and testing in order to enjoy full benefit of the management protocols.

He said management was multidisciplinary and involved commitment from both client and the caregivers. From de-stigmatization through adequate balanced diet to prompt treatment of the opportunists and highly active antiretroviral therapy when due, he noted that great strides had been made. To my relish and relief, he added that they was still no cure. To your relief and relish he listed preventive measures which to me actually looked simple. The only effective vaccine, he chided, was knowledge.

He checked the time, he had five minutes more. Some fun stuff would not harm his article, he decided.

He would sign out by comparing me to diabetes, another disease that required a lifelong management. People presently got their antiretroviral drugs free, he asserted, while diabetics had to buy their drugs. Again, those with me were encouraged to eat whereas the diabetics occasionally faced some dietary restrictions. He also noted that diabetes could also kill rapidly if left unchecked. Diabetes was usually overt clinically engendering early diagnosis unlike me. Again, he added, one could work hard at getting or not getting me and succeed at it, whereas one did not really decide his fate when it came to diabetes. Conclusively, he vented, his HIV, was better off managed well than diabetes contrary to most views.

He also talked of "long term non-progressors" in HIV were patients did not progress or progressed rather slowly. He wished he was one of such. With a word of caution that this should not seed another misconception, he also wrote about a select group of people in The Gambia and Kenya he'd read off the internet. The so called "Highly Exposed Persistently Seronegatives" (HEPS). These have had repeated exposure and have so far not been infected.

Then he made mention of some people in the US going to parties to actually seek HIV infection. These "gift" receivers actually actively sought the "gift" givers—the gift being me!

The burden of untreated patients was still unacceptable, he lamented. He prophesied that newer generation of antiretroviral drugs would hopefully be unveiled with improved toxicity profiles and ultimately, a cure. Better preventive measures would be discovered and ultimately a vaccine, he wished. Meanwhile, he warned, a constant invisible laser was beamed at every one. It required educated actions to avoid these trigger happy viral tentacles. I couldn't agree more with him. He was done with me on paper. He had a long life ahead to deal with me. With his knowledge, he had the upper hand.

*   *   *

As he proceeded to answer another question, I shifted my attention to somewhere in my gloomy past. A voice singing in sorrow:

"Today is me, tomorrow someone else, it's me and you, we've got (to) stand and fight, we shed a light in the fight against AIDS, let's come on out. Let's stand together (to) fight AIDS."

It was *Philly Lutaaya,* a Ugandan musician whom I'd knocked out years ago. I remembered little *Nkosi* and other unsung heroes of your fight, fright and flight—affected, infected and infested, funny enough, I felt a tinge of guilt.

With this memoir, I wash my guilt. I am through.

Chapter Four

AFRAID

There have been carrying me about. The widow tilling the farmland to feed her hunger prone children, the driver who has traversed the width and breadth of the country behind wheels atop women, the drunk army recruit in the barrack, the neonate in the neonatal intensive care unit, a president of a federal republic, the big time prostitute that serviced the loins of a Senator last night, the patient whom you transfused yesteryear without adequate blood screening, the fifth wife whose husband has four other wives, your boyfriend, fiend actually, who happens to have another girlfriend, the girl you are wooing, the armed robber who raped a girl at gun point, the medical officer who had a needle stick injury, the revered reverend Father who did not respect his vow of celibacy and the homosexual across the street—the list is by no means exhaustive and it is growling, growing and gnawing when it shouldn't. Some know, some don't, but I know. Some are doing the right thing about it; others are not. I am keen on the path each chooses.

The health system needs a drop of blood to identify and help them, but few are willing to part with the sample. Bit by bit, I am taking them. It will soon be so obvious that even the market woman can make a tentative diagnosis.

From this limelight of iniquitous fame I have watched the ark built against me with a good foundation collapse because they have worked hard on everything but the roof. And it's raining on hats and rugs, cats and dogs. I am the rain and I have thunder and lightning at my disposal. The weatherman occasionally gets me right but most people turn a deaf ear. These same guys have been busy scooping out water under no roof while I take out canoodles from the human race in oodles of puddles. They have so many scoopers and scoop efficiently but as they start moping, the drizzle comes to promise torrential rains, typhoons and hurricanes that drive home the meaning of public health terminologies like epidemic, endemic and pandemic.

What are they not getting right? They start studying hard and discover the cause of the drenched floor is primarily the rain. That did not need hard studying, did it? They ask questions like "what is rain?" "Where does it come from?" One thing they still haven't got right. No scooping can be that effective. I tell you. If they get the roofs right, the floor can be taken care of. Even the smallest of mops will suffice. How do they get it right?

I am not saying I will stop myself overnight, but I guarantee I will spark the young brains that will dispatch me to the quietude of retirement. An elevator or a lift is what takes you up. That it also takes you down doesn't change its name. I am here to stem my tides. I am still HIV.

My pseudonym *Homo Invitus* roughly translates to Human Invited. I could have gone by any other name. When they found me, they somehow knew I was human invited. It was a name not borne out of love but hate, not given by parents but by science freaks. People have continued in this inviting manner. I am not the way, the truth and the light but everyone most hear my name, accept and believe that I exist to do what I do to stand a fair chance of escaping my wrath. In this gospel of mine, innocence is no excuse, not even for your unborn child.

I am willing to part with the roofing technology hoping you numskulls will not disregard my proposal. I will challenge and change the forecasted weather. Yes, I will augment Whaler's efforts. Reason: Africa was a miss-hit.

AFRAID is a term I coined for an initiative to release my pressure on Africa—Mother Africa, as you fondly call it. I set out to attack a different world entirely and Africa got caught in the crossfire. Far from the literary afraid, it is an intrepid acronym for *Africa* from *AIDS*. With commitment, it is an achievable goal.

After envisaging my *MIST* theory, I surmised that only a sustainable low resource means, piggybacked on existing infrastructures, can achieve respite from me. The factors militating against Africa included the triad of disease, ignorance and poverty (DIP). I increased the first, further deepening the dip, now I intend to reduce the second to create a new balance. I have also noted with dismay, that it is in your nature to allow the bricks to set before trying to bend it into shape. This does not work for me.

AFRAID is a vaccine that has always been there. It's a recovery, not a discovery. It uses Afraid Initiative Mantra (AIM) (vide infra) to effectively mentor-immunize sub-Saharan Africa, and indeed the world from me. I should be given the Nobel Prize for physiology for this.

My solution starts when you bring a child into this world. Tell it about me, before the brick sets! It's as simple as that.

Your kindergarten and nursery school systems should be commissioned to make your children know me—at least recite my initials. As they become conversant with basic "ABC . . ." and "123 . . ." in primary schools, they should memorize baseline information like the following staircase of factual phrases:

"HIV and AIDS"
"Know your status"
"Ignorance spreads HIV."
"HIV causes but is not AIDS."
"Hoarding HIV does not Halt HIV."
"I will not be ignorant of HIV and AIDS."
"HIV and AIDS are preventable and treatable."

In the second half of elementary schools, they should be able to recite the *AIM*. They should be taught my toll, the numbers, the pains and the costs inflicted.

In junior secondary schools, they should be taught the tenets of my *AIM* in details to ensure compliance.

As a home cell, routine annual family screening and education should be emphasized.

At all levels of education, HIV/AIDS clubs and competitions should be encouraged by adequate funding.

By the way (in the way rather), I will have you know that *MANTRA* is short for *Mother Africa Novel Ten Regime Agenda*. Mother Africa huh . . . it sounds good. I keep with the lingo, since my epidemiology has declared me African.

My mantra should appear on billboards continent wide. It should be recited like a Muslim scholar does the Koran and quoted like the Christian Pastor does the Bible.

For the general public too, places where I am easily accessible like prostituting zones, should be cautioned with *zebra crossings* and messages like:

"SLOW DOWN; HIV CROSSING."
"THE FEDERAL GOVERNMENT WARNS THAT YOU CAN GET HIV TODAY."
"A DANGEROUS TERRAIN, IF YOU MOST DRIVE; DRIVE BELOW CONDOM KM/H!"

I want this *AIM* entrenched in school curricular; it should constitute a giveaway question in every school graduation exam as well as employment interviews. The first compulsory question in the senior school certificate examination should predictably read: "*As relates to HIV-AIDS, discuss the AIM.*"

I am not being overbearing here. I need you to simply ingrain me in your offspring through an existing educational system. If I am not in their minds, I can always find my way into their bloodstream—your choice. Remember I am not fame hunting. I am already famous. I changed medicine overnight. I filled whole chapters of medical texts, changed the fundamental dogma of molecular physiology with my reverse transcriptase enzyme. I constitute a new infectious disease specialty. Volumes are being written about me requiring yearly updates, as a plethora of theories are proven and speculations thrown out. I ushered a new modus operandi. Some malignancies and organisms depend on me to wrought violence they never dreamt of. I allied and bolstered them. And now I am allying to bolster you with this lexical universal pre and post—exposure prophylaxis. I was forced to become a common enemy wreaking havoc, an enemy that threw the world into turmoil, and I am here to save it again. How famous can you get? If I were to be awarded the peace prize from Stockholm, it'd be less controversial than Barack Obama's.

*   *   *

Before I give you the AI*M*, some pertinent facts need to be highlighted as governing baseline. You may want to look up the obscure medical terminologies. And mind not my unadorned lyrics, I never went to college. I picked up the language from my clientele and those brainy physicians counselling and managing them. So the literati should transcribe the message down to the illiterate strata. Tell them to remember:

I do not arise from nothing. Any index case has another definite source case and other probable contacts.

In every polygamous home, my being positive in a parent constitutes an "endemic" that can degenerate into a pandemic if not identified and tackled immediately. While polygamy is moral, *it is not easy to vouch for each of the say four people living together.*

Antiretroviral drugs prevent my transmission from mother to child; behavioural modifications like abstinence and being faithful, consistent and correct usage of condoms prevent my transmission. *Believe me I am a one hundred percent preventable disaster.*

Many people do not know their status, hence the clear possibility of pre and post-seroconversion dissemination.

Intentional spread is also being rumoured.

Some beliefs and claims such as the sex with a virgin cure fallacy are still rife and constitute another setback in the fight against me.

Many people are still learning the hard way about me. *They get to know I really exist only when I have been found in them.*

Many of the "brief illness" you hear in obituaries are actually caused by me. Due to stigmatization, I still don't have a face. This makes me harder to control.

My association with Africa is unquestionably becoming more fearsome. It is perpetuated by a vicious DIP (disease, ignorance and poverty) circle yet to be broken in the depth of indebted sub-Saharan Africa.

Some practicing clinicians are of the opinion that my toll is being under quoted in some areas for socio-political reasons.

People are still cheated with supposed cures.

HIV causes but is not synonymous with AIDS.

I have seen many a husband living secretly with me, on drugs without the wife/wives knowing and vice versa too!

They are people living *with* me and people living *on* me. The later usurp funds meant to control me thereby hampering management of the former.

Traditionally, the first three letters of the alphabet: Abstinence, Being faithful and Condom has been used in adult prevention education. The child's largely empty, albeit sponge—like mind is capacious and is targeted with the alphabet's first ten letters. These should roof the Noah's ark you've been building against my flood and create a fortress that I will respect. After all I brokered this truce. I am no recidivist.

Down from Sinai; behold my ten tablets AIM commandments, with scribbling spaces provided for your brainstorming on implementing each. Pick a pen, here is paper; write away forever, the pain and caper I brought. If you got an e-copy, meditate on the spaces provided.

Actively Accept People Living With AIDS (PLWA); Assist the Affected too. Actively Avoid Alcohol Abuse.

Be there for them, don't Beware or Be away, but Be aware and Be tested.

Criminalize stigmatization and People Living On AIDS (PLOA). Ensure Client's Consent and Compassionate Confidentiality.

Drugs constitute only one aspect of management. Do TLC for those commencing them. And Do no Drug. *(DO TLC: Directly Observed Therapy Long Course; should also simply mean Do Tender Loving Care.)*

Educate Every age group on stopping the Epidemic especially in sub-Saharan Africa. *(Use contemporary ABC. Apply only Abstinence in primary school, Bring Being faithful to bear in junior secondary school and crown Condom usage in senior secondary school with emphasis still placed on the earlier lessons.)*

Feed only Facts, Fight and Foil Fallacies about HIV/

AIDS.

Give cash and kind to the cause. Garner support from Government and Non Governmental organization.

Help negative remain negative and Help positive live positively. HAART should be accompanied by Hearty meals.

I.V. drug users needle exchange programs. Institute risk management and Instil standard post exposure protocols.

Join AFRAID, Jilt and Jettison HIV/AIDS from Africa. *(If you know your status, you have joined AFRAID already.)*

An *AFRAID* compliant continent is an achievable goal. If adopted, the storm and flood will pass and awaken you to the rainbow of the possibility of a world without me. With this mnemonic memoir, I have dared you in so many words, told you what I have done, how I came to be, how I work and how I can be undone by simple sustainable means. I have even conscripted you into writing out your script on stopping me into my own scripture . . . from my *genesis* and *exodus* from *numbers* of *judges* and *kings*; I *chronicle* the *lamentations* that *mark* my *acts* to the *revelation* of a ceasefire.

If I were a Muslim, I'd be Allah's prophet, if I were Catholic I'd be canonized by the Holy See and if I belonged to the old African religion, I'd be a god.

But I am only a virus tied to killing but tired of killing.

So I ask Africa from Cape to Cairo. What are you going to do with the *AIM* content of my memoir? Will countries adopt legislatures to educate children about the AIM from the womb to the tomb? Will I appear on every question paper from primary to tertiary schools? Will the stigma jinx be broken? Will a new map of awareness and action be unveiled to reflect the changes I scribbled these pages for? Or would you rather continue the hide and seek game with me playing the seeker while you preys pay with the sicker part?

Here, I have offered my hands and you wield the cuffs. Grab this chance, Africa. It may be your only chance. For sure, it's the only time I will come to your aid and not give you your feared plural AIDS. If you work at it, I will remain truly *not* yours, HIV, the causative bug of the truly life sapping, AIDS.

I am neither God's blessing bliss nor Satan's blazing blitz. It's farewell to terrorism. I have written myself off the continent. Read and rid me off the globe!

The end.

Authors Note

I am only the editor.

I thank those who will make sure someone else benefits from this "hearing from the horse's mouth." If you've just gone through it like any other novella, you need to go back to it as a document and get the worth of these words. Make a commitment list in the spaces provided on how you intend to obey the AIM commandments. Do this with your family, class, patients, peers, and constitute an implementation committee. Personally review each commitment every six months. You can ask an artist to design a framed billboard with the AIM for teaching. A miniature version is suggested overleaf.

It is true, AIDS, even in the presence of HIV, is one hundred percent preventable in most cases, but we tend to start out late. Now is not too early. We've got work to do. Prevention is better than cure, that's elementary. How much better is prevention when and where they is no cure. Bring the *AIM* into your home to keep HIV and AIDS out.

Whose birth day is it; you are reading the ideal present. Proprietors, here is edification for your tutors from kindergarten to high schools. Physicians, here is a recommended tool for wide scale prevention and management of HIV, be sure to include it in your prescription for both positive and negative clients. Ministries of health, here is a societal vaccine, distribute it. Information Ministries, here is an all important information, disseminate it. And to the youth, here is to your future, toast to it.

Know your status today and do the right thing about it. That is the only way to kick-start the new beginning, the only way to salvage the impending covert wreckage posed by this viral genie.

You are hereby immunized with the attendant onus of immunizing a neighbour.

Our future without HIV/AIDS is possible.

Afraid Initiative Mantra (Aim)

A. Actively Accept People Living With AIDS (PLWA); Assist the Affected too. Actively Avoid Alcohol Abuse.

B. Be there for them, don't Beware or Be away, but Be aware and Be tested.

C. Criminalize stigmatization and People Living On AIDS (PLOA). Ensure Client's Consent and Compassionate Confidentiality.

D. Drugs constitute only one aspect of management. Do TLC for those commencing them. And Do no Drug.

E. Educate Every age group on stopping the Epidemic especially in sub-Saharan Africa.

F. Feed only Facts, Fight and Foil Fallacies about HIV/AIDS.

G. Give cash and kind to the cause. Garner support from Government and Non Governmental organization.

H. Help negative remain negative and Help positive live positively. HAART should be accompanied by Hearty meals.

I. I.V. drug users needle exchange programs. Institute risk management and Instil standard post exposure protocols.

J. Join AFRAID, Jilt and Jettison HIV/AIDS from Africa.

www.ingramcontent.com/pod-product-compliance
Lightning Source LLC
Chambersburg PA
CBHW061217280526
45784CB00006B/2516